TABLE OF CONTENTS

Judgment Not Included
The Mindset of the Unbalanced
©Copyright 2013 by Dr. Leland Benton

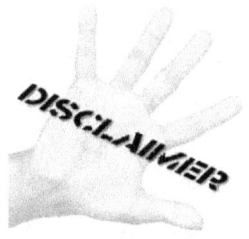

DISCLAIMER AND TERMS OF USE AGREEMENT:

(Please Read This Before Using This Book)

This information is for educational and informational purposes only. The content is not intended to be a substitute for any professional advice, diagnosis, or treatment.

The author and publisher of this book and the accompanying materials have used their best efforts in preparing this book.

The author and publisher make no representation or warranties with respect to the accuracy, applicability, fitness, or completeness of the contents of this book. The information contained in this book is strictly for educational purposes. Therefore, if you wish to apply ideas contained in this book, you are taking full responsibility for your actions.

The author and publisher disclaim any warranties (express or implied), merchantability, or fitness for any particular purpose. The author and publisher shall in no event be held liable to any party for any direct, indirect, punitive, special, incidental or other consequential damages arising directly or indirectly from any use of this material, which is provided "as is", and without warranties. As always, the advice of a competent legal, tax, accounting, medical or other professional should be sought where applicable.

The author and publisher do not warrant the performance, effectiveness or applicability of any sites listed or linked to in this book. All links are for information purposes only and are not warranted for content, accuracy or any other implied or explicit purpose. No part of this may be copied, or changed in any format, or used in any way other than what is outlined within this course under any circumstances. Violators will be prosecuted.

Introduction – The Mindset of the Unbalanced

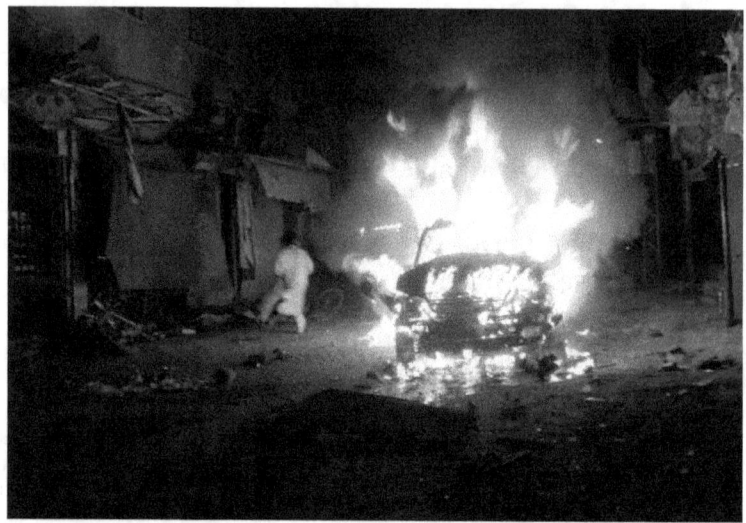

Agence France-Presse — Getty Images
A suicide bombing in Peshawar, Pakistan, this month. Innocent Muslims are killed by radical Muslims in the Middle East weekly.

In this book, I will examine the mindset of the unbalanced; what makes them tick, why they commit the heinous crimes that they do; are insanity and/or psychological issues grounds for defense and more.

It is becoming commonplace for the evening news to report some of the most terrible crimes committed by unbalanced people. As I write this book, the bombing of the Boston Marathon has taken place. Sandy Hook Elementary School killings have occurred; the murder of moviegoers in Aurora, Colorado takes it sad place in history; the shooting of Congresswoman Gabrielle Gifford has occurred and many more.

Every day, some type of crime is committed by unbalanced people and the debate rages as to what consequences are justified for their actions.

I have been a behavioral scientist for over 32-years. I am also Chief Forensics Investigator for ForensicsNation for over 32-years and in my role as an investigator, I have busted and caused the capture of over 1100 criminals. In both my professional roles, I am highly qualified to write this book fro I know the criminal mind, the mind of the unbalanced and much more as I profile them and provide insight into their insidious intents.

First, read the following article that sparked me to write this book…

Judgment Not Included

http://www.nytimes.com/2013/04/28/opinion/sunday/friedman-judgment-not-included.html?nl=todaysheadlines&emc=edit_th_20130428&_r=1&

By THOMAS L. FRIEDMAN
Published: April 27, 2013

AS police investigators peel away the layers of the Boston Marathon bombing, there are two aspects of this unfolding story to which I want to react: the mind-set of the alleged bombers and the role of the Internet in shaping it. Important news about both was contained in a single Washington Post article on Tuesday.

"The 19-year-old suspect in the Boston Marathon bombings has told interrogators that the American wars in Iraq and Afghanistan motivated him and his brother to carry out the attack, according to U.S. officials familiar with the interviews," The Post reported. The officials said, "Dzhokhar and his older brother, Tamerlan Tsarnaev ... do not appear to have been directed by a foreign terrorist organization. Rather, the officials said, the evidence so far suggests they were 'self-radicalized' through Internet sites and U.S. actions in the Muslim world. Dzhokhar Tsarnaev has specifically cited the U.S. war in Iraq, which ended in December 2011 with the removal of the last American forces, and the war in Afghanistan."

This is a popular meme among radical Muslim groups, and, to be sure, some Muslim youths were deeply angered by the U.S. interventions in the Middle East. The brothers Tsarnaev may have been among them.

But what in God's name does that have to do with planting a bomb at the Boston Marathon and blowing up innocent people? It is amazing to me how we've come to accept this non sequitur and how easily we've allowed radical Muslim groups and their apologists to get away with it.

A simple question: If you were upset with U.S. wars in Iraq and Afghanistan, why didn't you go out and build a school in Afghanistan to strengthen that community or

6

get an advanced degree to strengthen yourself or become a math teacher in the Muslim world to help its people be less vulnerable to foreign powers? Dzhokhar claims the Tsarnaev brothers were so upset by something America did in a third country that they just had to go to Boylston Street and blow up people who had nothing to do with it (some of whom could have been Muslims), and too often we just nod our heads rather than asking: What kind of sick madness is this?

It's a double non sequitur when it comes from Muslim youths who lived and studied in America, where, if you're upset about something, you have many ways to express your opposition and have an impact — from organizing demonstrations to publishing articles to running for office. In fact, an American guy named Barack, whose grandfather was a Muslim, did just that. And he's now president of the United States, a job he's used to unwind the wars in Iraq and in Afghanistan.

Moreover, some 70,000 people, most of them Muslims, have been killed by other Muslims in the Syrian civil war, which the U.S. had nothing to do with — although many Muslims are now begging us to intervene to stop it. And every week innocent Muslims are blown up by Muslim suicide bombers in Pakistan and Iraq — every week. Thousands of them have been maimed and killed in attacks so nihilistic that the bombers don't even bother to give their names or make demands. Yet this does not appear to have moved the brothers Tsarnaev one iota.

Why is that? We surely must not tar all of Islam in this. Having lived in the Muslim world, I know how unfair that would be. But we must ask a question only Muslims can answer: What is going on in your community that a critical number of your youth believes that every American military action in the Middle East is intolerable and justifies a violent response, and everything Muslim extremists do to other Muslims is ignorable and calls for mostly silence?

As for the role that Web sites apparently played in the "self-radicalization" of the two Chechen brothers, it is yet another reminder that the Internet is a digital river that carries incredible sources of wisdom and hate along the same current. It's all there together. And our kids and citizens usually interact with this flow nakedly, with no supervision.

So more people are more directly exposed to more raw information and opinion every day from everywhere. As such, it is more important than ever that we build the internal software, the internal filters, into every citizen to sift out fact from fiction in this electronic torrent, which offers so much information that has never been touched by an editor, a censor or a libel lawyer. That's why, when the Internet first emerged and you had to connect via a modem, I used to urge that modems sold in America come with a warning label from the surgeon general, like cigarettes. It would read: "Attention: Judgment not included."

And that's why the faster, more accessible and ultramodern the Internet becomes, the more all the old-fashioned stuff matters: good judgment, respect for others who are different and basic values of right and wrong.

Those you can't download. They have to be uploaded, the old-fashioned way, by parents around the dinner table, by caring but demanding teachers at school and by responsible spiritual leaders in a church, synagogue, temple or mosque. Somewhere, somehow, that did not happen, or stopped happening, with the brothers Tsarnaev.

*****

As the above article indicates, the Muslim community remains silent as to the radicalization of its youth and every time something like the Boston Marathon bombing occurs, they hunker down within their communities expecting the worst but hoping for the best.

Is it fair to ask why? These Muslims are American citizens for the most part, and I am sure they are just as traumatized as other Americans at the senseless violence here and in the Arab world but are they doing anything about it?

The above author of the article is justified to ask the question but I disagree with his indictment of the Internet just as I disagree with the gun debate to restrict firearms. Both are band-aid approaches to the problem and it is this problem I will address in this book.

I first will begin with a brief lesson in behavioral science where I want you to understand how the human mind operates; the actual mechanism of the mind, and its associated functions.

I then want to delve into the subject of why the unbalanced do what they do and then address the defense of using psychological issues as a valid excuse for the unbalanced.

It is important that you learn how to spot an unbalanced person and also how to protect yourself in today's world and I have added both of these chapters in this book.

This book is part of my Cyber Crime/ Cyber Forensics series of books:

Confessions of a Child Predator
http://www.amazon.com/dp/B007BB97KU
Child Watch
http://www.amazon.com/dp/B0095K1P3M
Cyber-Daters Beware
http://www.amazon.com/dp/B006J9T4NA
Cyber Protect Your Business
http://www.amazon.com/dp/B0095JEAYY
ForensicsNation Bushwhacker Program
http://www.amazon.com/dp/B007I9AHVS
ForensicsNationsStore.com Catalog
http://ForensicsNationStore.com
Protecting Yourself from Cyber Crime
http://www.amazon.com/dp/B0095J3EIW
Stealing You
http://www.amazon.com/dp/B00778TT6E
The Mind Of a Con Man

http://www.amazon.com/dp/B00CO2BQHI
Was Sandy Hook a Hoax?
http://www.amazon.com/dp/B00BFSM8IS
Why Women Should Not Use Online Dating Services
http://www.amazon.com/dp/B006J9EMH8
You Can Run But You Cannot Hide
http://www.amazon.com/dp/B006JLVZC6

My goal with this series of books is to provide my readers with concise information on how to protect themselves from the inherent risks that they confront daily.

The responsibility of protecting yourself rests with YOU! Not law enforcement and not any outside entity...but YOU!

Once you take this responsibility to heart, protecting you and your loved ones is not as difficult as it may appear.

It is my goal to demonstrate the techniques I teach in my seminars and online webinars so that you too can be empowered and confident.

So., let's begin to unravel the puzzle...

Chapter 1 - Laying A Proper Foundation

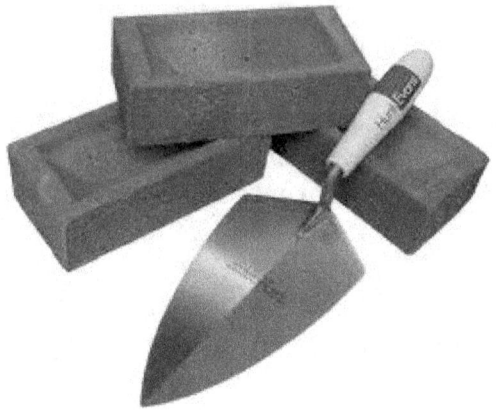

In all of my "Why" series of books, I will provide the following discourse on the Human Mind in order to lay a proper foundation to what I am about to teach.

The Mechanism of the Human Mind

Which Comes First - the Body or the Mind?

(the most important concept in all of talk therapy)

Understanding the Body - Mind Connection

For thousands of years, we have known there is a body – mind connection. Until now though, we have not known what this connection is. What it it? Time. The body and the mind each have their own sense of time. Their own clocks so to speak. Therapy works only when these two clocks are in sync.

| Body First
Person | Body – Mind
in sync | Mind First
Person |

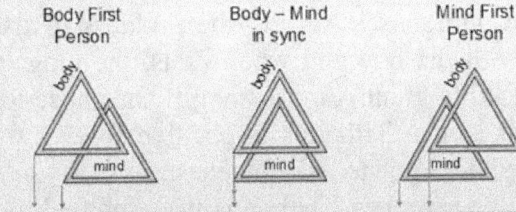

Prior to the fall of man into sin as described in the Garden of Eden, man's spirit was hooked to God's infinite spirit. There was no death because God's spirit is infinite. Man is the only animal on earth that shares the eternality nature of God. The subject of eternal life has been a heated topic of man from the beginning of our existence.

In Greek mythology, there's a story about a mortal youth named Tithonus. Aurora, the goddess of dawn, fell in love with the boy and when Zeus, the king of the gods, promised to grant Aurora any gift she chose for her lover, she asked that Tithonus might live forever. But, in her haste she forgot to ask for eternal youth, so when Zeus granted her request, Tithonus was doomed to an eternity of perpetual aging as a grouchy old man… forever.

In the movie "Highlander," Angus McLeod was born in 1518 as an immortal being. He could not die and to me, the best part of the movie was the depiction of this immortal's agony here on earth as he watched everything he loved die forcing him to begin his life over and over again. He saw all of the ugliness, which man had caused over four centuries. He witnessed the Spanish Inquisition, Waterloo, the atrocities of the Third Reich, and more. He saw the slavery and bigotry of the eighteenth century, the slaughter of the Native American tribes after the Civil War. This man's life was a living Hell!

There is a very big difference between the ways our feeble minds picture eternal life versus God's idea of eternal life. Our understanding comes from Quantum Physics and is limited within the Time-Space Continuum.

Life is your spirit, but the soul of man has usurped the spirit's position and psychology is now forced to define "how" we live our lives based on the animating force of the soul instead of the spirit. As I said previously, the soul has usurped the spirit's place as our animating force. Let's discuss this now.

❖ **Body First Person** - When the body becomes our life, we live as animals.
❖ **Body-Mind In Sync** - When the soul becomes our life, we live as rebels and fugitives in a life of desires, emotions, and will (consuming entities). This is the position of mankind today!
❖ **Mind First Person** - But when we come to live our life in the mind/spirit and by the spirit, though we still use our soul's faculties just as we do our physical faculties, they are now the servants of the spirit.

If you live as a consuming entity, you will always lose. In other words, to get, you must give - you must sacrifice! Have you ever wondered why you have so many anxieties, phobias, worries and fears? The reality of this world is evil. So what is reality? I will tell you. This is reality:

"Life without war is impossible either in nature or in grace. The basis of physical, mental, moral and spiritual life is antagonism. Health is the balance between physical life and external nature, and it is maintained only by sufficient vitality on the inside against things on the

15

outside. Everything outside my physical life is designed to put me to death. Things, which keep me going when I am alive, disintegrate me when I am dead. If I have enough fighting power, I produce the balance of health.

The same is true of mental life. If I want to maintain a vigorous mental life, I have to fight, and in that way the mental balance called thought is produced. Morally it is the same. Everything that does not partake of the nature of virtue is the enemy of virtue in me, and it depends on what moral caliber I have whether I overcome and produce virtue (GOOD CHARACTER). Immediately I fight, I am moral in that particular. No man is virtuous because he cannot help it; virtue (character) is acquired.

- ❖ Psychology only studies the observable aspects of the mind and discounts the unseen or intangible aspects of the human mind.
- ❖ Behavioral science attempts to study the intangible aspects of the human mind…why you do the things you do and more importantly why you don't do what you should do.
- ❖ There is no such thing as commercial psychology versus personal psychology. The mind uses the same mechanism to evaluate all types of relationships.
- ❖ Everything we do revolves around relationships. We relate to our environment, our friends, family, co-workers, other people and even our pets. We are social animals.

The Mechanism of the Human Mind

Belief Systems + Thought + Delight = Action/Behavior/Conduct

Conscious Mind

5-senses:
Sight
Hearing
Taste
Touch
Smell
ESP (women only)

Subconscious Mind

Intellect:
Experiential
Empirical

DEW:
Desires, Emotions and Will

The Human Psyche Differences Between Genders

The female psyche operates on emotional, spiritual, physical and intellectual planes
The male psyche operates only on the intellectual and physical planes.

Here is an exercise you might find weird but it demonstrates the power of the human mind.

Fi yuo cna raed tihs, yuo hvae a sgtrane mnid too. Cna yuo raed tihs? Olny 55 plepoe out of 100 can. I cdnuolt blveiee taht I cluod aulaclty uesdnatnrd waht I was rdanieg. The phaonmneal pweor of the hmuan mnid, aoccdrnig to a rscheearch at Cmabrigde Uinervtisy, it dseno't mtaetr in waht oerdr the ltteres in a wrod are, the olny iproamtnt tihng is taht the frsit and lsat ltteer be in the rghit pclae. The rset can be a taotl mses and you can sitll raed it whotuit a pboerlm. Tihs is bcuseae the huamn mnid deos not raed ervey lteter by istlef, but the wrod as a wlohe. Azanmig huh? Yaeh and I awlyas tghuhot slpeling was ipmorantt!

You might have found it somewhat unusual that you could probably read the jumbled mess above. Actually over half the people that see this exercise can decipher the words at the same speed of reading as if the words were not jumbled.

It is important to note that the human mind thinks in packages...concepts rather than individual ideas.

Your eyes see each letter but the mind looks at the whole word instead. As you read, the mind looks at the first and last letter only. Remember this; the mind sees the beginning and end. We will talk about this later...

If you were to listen to an orchestra, your ear listens to every note from every instrument but a trained ear can actually pick out individual instruments from the whole sound as the mind hears the whole symphony.

How does this apply to you?

Learning to observe means going beyond the mind's natural ability to only read the first and last letters of a word!

It is training the mind to see all the letters, not just the eye but the mind!

Truisms About the Human Mind

- ❖ Pain vs. Pleasure – people are more motivated to avoid pain than seek pleasure.
- ❖ A person that is suffering depression will seek relief (notice I didn't say cure) before they seek happiness.
- ❖ The human mind cannot tell the difference between fantasy and reality.
- ❖ The human mind gravitates to the desires, emotions and will of its psyche. People crave entertainment so fantasy dominates their existences.
- ❖ The human mind is easily distracted! You can either be the cause of these distractions or other stimuli will be the cause but rest assured people WILL BE distracted because the human mind is gullible.

The human mind responds quickly to these three forms of stimuli

- ❖ Sex
- ❖ Humor
- ❖ FEAR

But the greatest of them all is FEAR!

BTW – on the positive side we have faith, hope, love, but the greatest of these *is* LOVE.

Fear usually takes the form of what is called "Scarcity Thought"

You are afraid that someone will have what you feel belongs to you or that others will have more "stuff" than you.

❖ The subconscious mind is often referred to as the "heart," and is the control mechanism the body uses to store our beliefs.

❖ **These beliefs are stored as pictures in our "hearts" and create frequencies in our bodies.**

❖ We know that the optimum human frequency is a little below 7.83 hertz. To drop below this frequency brings on the onslaught of disease. To rise above it a person demonstrates psychic abilities.

❖ Harmful beliefs that cause unhealthy frequencies are the source of almost all problems - physical, mental, emotional.

❖ The subconscious mind creates a belief system, which we call "pictures of the heart."

❖ These pictures involve either visions, or dreams/fantasies.

❖ Science has discovered that the subconscious mind cannot distinguish between fantasy and reality.

*The subject of all dreams is the dreamer.
*Dreams are born in our desires, emotions and will.
*Dreamers believe in a belief system, which is fantasy.
*A life lived within a fantasy creates a feeling of self-centeredness, hopelessness and despair. In dreams everything is perfect.
*The subject of a vision is not the visionary but the world.
*Visions are born in the intellect.
*Visions are pictures of the future that have already been experienced in the heart of those who give it birth.
*Visionaries sacrifice themselves for the good of mankind.
*Visions have a moral quality that transcends the self-centered nature of dreams.
*By its very nature a vision launches a mission, a "cause-that-inspires."
*Visions create a sense of belonging.

❖ We act upon visions and/or dreams, using thought.
❖ Thought employs the intellect, in the case of visions, or the desires, emotions and the will, in the case of dreams.
❖ Intellectual thought relies on wisdom; emotional thought relies on the pursuit of pleasure, comfort and delight.
❖ Dreamers live within a facade; they create a false sense of worth using imaginary situations.

- ❖ Visionaries live within reality; they create change, within a framework of restraint, and intellectual thought.
- ❖ The world is made up of OPPOSITES, which is usually the corrupted version of the original. We have good and evil. We have love and lust!
- ❖ EVERYTHING YOU DO IS BECAUSE OF LOVE OR LUST. Learn to love because there are no crimes beyond forgiveness.

*Love is born in the intellect; lust is born in the DEW!
*Love is vision; lust is fantasy.
*Love restrains & sacrifices; lust is selfish
*Love is being one with someone or something
*Lust is being with someone or something.
*Visionaries love; dreamers lust!
*Visionaries do what is required; dreamers just do their best!

WHEN THERE IS NO HOPE OF LOVE DO WE ABANDON OURSELVES TO LUST?

Yes we do!

Pictures of the heart are your belief system.

- ❖ We animate these pictures into either fantasies, or visions.
- ❖ People do not appear to see the difference between the matter part of an organism and the life part, which animates it.

- ❖ We seem to think that the organism itself is life. In other words, it is not our outward appearance that is our life, but our inward existence.
- ❖ Life is what goes into the body. Death is what comes out.
- ❖ A person who lies is not a liar because he tells a lie. The lie is the manifested behavior of some subconscious belief system. The lie only demonstrates that the person is a liar…it is the effect.
- ❖ Except for love, the power of words inspired by a vision or fantasy is the most potent human force.

"Do you want to have or do you want to be?"

*For a dreamer: "Seeing is believing!"
*But they only see imaginary things that are not real!!
*This is why "The Secret" is WRONG!
*Say it and claim it is WRONG!
*Blab it and grab it IS WRONG!
*See it and be it IS WRONG!
Dreamers practice companionship – To be with someone or something!

VERY IMPORTANT:

1. Dreamers covet the object of their temptation, BUT they covet the temptation more so than the object itself because the temptation is the idol of their fantasy.
2. If there is a conflict between the conscious and subconscious mind, the subconscious mind always wins…ALWAYS!

23

3. All reaction occurs in the conscious mind; all interaction occurs in the subconscious mind. Fear is a "REACTION" to losing control.

For a visionary: "Believing is seeing!"

There are no SECRETS; there are only challenges to be conquered!

THIS IS NOT A SECRET: Putting a photo of a Ferrari on your refrigerator and seeing yourself driving it by employing the so-called law of attraction is pure BUPKES!!! Why? Because this is all occurring in the conscious mind and beliefs reside in the subconscious mind. How do you transfer something from the conscious mind to the subconscious mind and make it a belief system?

A Ferrari is the object of your temptation but what you covet most is the temptation of owning a Ferrari because the temptation is the idol of your fantasy.

It is all about ATTENTION & ACCEPTANCE!!!!! I have a $100 bill in my hand and I am willing to give it to you. But if you don't ACCEPT it then it is still in my hand. BELIEF SYSTEMS ARE CREATED BY ATTENTION & ACCEPTANCE!

John 1:12 But as many as received him, to them gave he **the right** to become children of God, *even* to them that believe on his name

Human things must be known to be loved; but divine things must be loved to be known.

BELIEVING IS SEEING!

Let's talk about goals...which of the following goals are good goals?

❖ To want to get married and have a wonderful, happy, loving marriage?
❖ To want to have children who are happy, successful, and loving?
❖ To have a successful, fulfilling and rewarding career?
❖ Is it a good goal to want to have fun, bonded, loving, and meaningful relationships with other people?

Which of the listed goals are good goals?   None of them!

You should never have anything for a goal that is not 100% under your control, AND each and every goal should be <u>motivated by love</u>.

Almost all goals that we have in our life are wrong.

Everything that we do, we do because of a goal we have.

When we get up in the morning, it's because of some goal that we have; we are hungry for breakfast, or we need to go to work.

If we go to the grocery store, it's because of some goal we have. If we are kind to people, it's because of some goal that we have.

Now we don't always know what they are, because a lot of these are subconscious goals.

The goals we have are the reasons for everything we do. But, do all of your goals involve only YOU?

Of course not!

And when the other person, or persons, in your goal do not perform, or act the way you want them to, then we become anxious and stressed.

When our goals get blocked, it creates anger, anxiety, and frustration. If we only have good goals, we will not experience anger or anxiety.

That's how you know, if you are living a wrongful goal. If the result is anger and frustration because your control was blocked and blocking your goal, then you had a wrongful goal. It may have been a fine and noble desire, but a wrongful goal.

Filters
We live in a society of consumerism and entertainment. In my previous books I have spoken reams about this subject. Instant gratification is paramount and today's technology delivers information and other stimuli in bucketfuls to the human mind. We have already spoken about filters that the human mind employs to weed out

what it determines to be irrelevant. This "irrelevancy" is different in every individual and many times is programmed into our minds subconsciously or without us knowing it. We have also spoken about the causes of these various filters such as environment, maturity, upbringing, culture, etc.

The one essential common element of all filters is that they are all ATTENTION diverters. We have spoken about attention earlier; what is very interesting is that filters are generally viewed as bad when some are really very good.

I had a friend, who lives in Chicago, fall on hard times and needed assistance. When I got to him he was living in a cheap hotel and had a room so small when you put the key in the door you broke the *window (I slay me)*. His room was about 50 feet from the Loop (the overhead train that circles around Chicago). The noise was deafening when the train went by, and it went by often, but my friend had filtered it out. Amazing, but when you thing about it, my friend really does hear the train but yet he pays no attention to it, so in actuality, it is like he doesn't hear it at all! So filters divert attention, and take away our focus; so let's talk about focus.

The Incredible Power of Focus
One of the more important points I have made has been the idea that you really do create your own life and your own reality. I know this idea has become a kind of personal growth cliché that many of us have heard over and over for years. Many people, after continuing to experience the same old ups and downs and personal dramas over many years, get to the point where they dismiss this idea as charming but useless -- or just plain

wrong. "If I'm creating this, then I'm certainly not doing it on purpose," they say. "It sure seems like this is HAPPENING to me, rather than that I'm creating it." They just assume that it's all BS because "this and this and this and this are going on for me, and I have no control over it, and anyone who thinks I'm creating this doesn't understand what I'm going through." Essentially, they are resigning themselves to becoming a victim of circumstances.

We live in a universe of infinite complexity and many forces -- way too many to keep track of -- operate on us. Yes, it is true that we are NOT in control of everything that happens, because we are not in control of most of those infinite other parts of the universe. In fact, the only thing you have total and complete control over is...YOUR OWN MIND. That is, if you learn how to exercise it.

Luckily, this one thing -- your mind -- that you do have control over gives you tremendous power. By exercising control over your mind, you can get the rest of those infinite other parts of the universe to begin to march in formation.

The person who says, "If I'm creating this, it certainly isn't on purpose," is right. They are not creating what is happening to them "on purpose." Who would purposely create failure, or bad relationships, or any other kind of suffering? You can only do something that is not good for you that is harmful to you, if you do it subconsciously. This means if you are creating something you don't want, you must be doing so subconsciously.

Your mind is running on automatic pilot, based on "software" (subconscious programming) installed when you were too young to know any better, by parents, teachers, friends, the media, and other experiences and influences. The key is to become more conscious, more aware...to get yourself off automatic pilot. Once you do this, you stop creating all the dramas and other garbage you don't want in your life.

How do you do this? One way is by remembering and using a very important piece of wisdom. What is this important piece of wisdom? I'm glad you asked.

It's the fact that whatever you focus on manifests as reality in your life.

You are always focusing on something, whether you are aware of it or not. If I spent some time with you, and heard your history, I could tell you what you are focusing on. How? By looking at the results you are getting in your life. The results you get are always the result of your focus.

The problem is this focus is usually not conscious focus; it's automatic or subconscious focus. We subconsciously focus on something we don't want, and then when we get it we feel like a victim and don't even stop to think that we created it in the first place. And what is more, we don't realize we could choose to create something completely different if we could only get out of the cycle of subconsciously focusing on something other than what we want.

If you have a significant negative emotional experience (say, for instance, a relationship in which you are abused or mistreated in some way), a part of you is going to say: "Okay, I get it. There are people out there who can and will hurt me. Relationships can be dangerous and painful. I have to watch out for these people [or sometimes,

29

relationships in general] and avoid them." Unfortunately, to watch out for them and avoid them, you have to focus your mind on "people who could hurt me," or "bad relationships," and that focus draws more of what you don't want to you...AND...actually makes these things you don't want (at least initially) attractive to you, so when they appear in your life you are drawn to them. This is why many people keep having one relationship after another with the same person, but in different bodies. This, of course, applies to everything, not just relationships. I'm just using relationships as an example.

Focusing on what you do not want, ironically, makes it happen. Focusing on not being poor makes you poor. Focusing on not making mistakes causes you to make mistakes. Focusing on not having a bad relationship creates bad relationships. Focusing on not being depressed makes you depressed. Focusing on not smoking makes you want to smoke. And so on. I think you get the idea. The mind will create what you focus on both GOOD and BAD!!!

The truth is your mind cannot tell the difference between something you think about or focus on that you DO want, and something you think about or focus on but do NOT want. The mind is a goal-seeking mechanism, and an extremely effective one at that. Already, all the time, it is elegantly and precisely creating exactly what you focus on. You are already a World Champion Expert at creating whatever you focus on. You couldn't get any better at it, and you don't need to get any better at it.

When you focus on anything, your mind says: "Okay, we can do that," and starts figuring out how to do it. It doesn't ask whether you're focusing on it because you want it or because you do not want it. It ALWAYS assumes you want what you focus on and then it goes and makes it happen. The more frequent and the more intense the focus, the faster and more completely you will create what you have focused on, which is why intense negative experiences create intense focus on what you do not want, and tend to make you re-create what you don't want, over and over.

Most of the time, for most people, all the focusing and thinking is going by at warp speed, on automatic, without much, if any, conscious intention. Your job is to learn how to direct this power by consciously directing your focus to the outcomes you want. Once you do, everything changes. This does, however, take some work, because at first you have to swim upstream against the current of your old, unconscious habits, and the current can be swift and strong. Trained observation actually teaches you to focus on what you want.

First, you have to discover all the things you focus on that you do not want, and I'm willing to bet there are quite a few -- way more than you think. To the degree you're getting what you don't want, you are focusing, albeit subconsciously, on what you don't want.

Spend some time over the next few weeks making a list of all the things you do NOT want as you notice yourself thinking about them.

Second, you have to get very clear about what you DO want. Then, you have to examine each of the things you want and be sure they are not just something you do NOT want in disguise. For instance, saying "I want a relationship where I am treated well" would not even be an issue if you had not had relationships where you were not treated well, and even in making this seemingly positive statement you are focusing on not wanting to be mistreated. Saying "I want a reliable car" wouldn't even come up if you weren't focusing on the fact that you don't want a car that breaks down and needs a lot of repairs.

After you've sorted out the things you habitually focus on that you do not want, and know what you do want, you have to begin to notice each time you think about an outcome you do not want, and consciously change your thinking, right in that moment, so you are instead focusing on what you do want.

Remember, you do NOT have to avoid things to be happy and get what you want. The urge to avoid something is a result of having had a negative emotional experience regarding that thing, and trying to avoid things requires you to focus on them, which tells your brain to create them. Not good.

You will be surprised how often you are thinking about what you do not want, how difficult it is to catch yourself doing it every time, and -- most of all – how difficult it is to switch your thinking to what you DO want. There is a strong momentum to keep thinking about that thing you want to avoid. As I said, the current is strong and swift, especially at first.

The solution? Practice, practice, practice. Persistence, persistence, persistence!!!

It's a very good idea to write down what you want, very specifically, so that your Fairy Godmother, were she to read it, would know exactly what to give you without any additional explanation.

Then, read what you have written to yourself, preferably out loud, several times a day, while seeing yourself, in your mind, already having what you want.

Believing is seeing and not the other way around as the world teaches you!

The more emotion you can bring to it, the better. Then, take whatever action is available to begin moving toward what you want. A good time to do this reading and visualizing is when you first wake up and before you go to bed.

I know this is work. Do it anyway. There is a price for everything, and this is the price you must pay to get what you want. Be prepared to pay it. It will be worth it, I promise. And be prepared to pay for a while before you get results. Stick with it.

Another way to change your focus is to ask questions. As an example, I'll ask you one right now. What did you have for breakfast this morning? To answer this question (even to just internally process the question), you had to shift your focus from whatever your mind was focused on (hopefully, to what I am teaching) to today's breakfast.

This means that to change your focus, all you have to do is...ask yourself a question!

It also means you better be careful what questions you ask yourself. Good questions include "How can I get X?" "How can I do X?" "How can I be X?" By asking these kinds of questions, you get your mind to focus on what you want to have, do, or be. Then, your mind takes over and answers the question...solves the problem...and creates what you want. You just have to provide the focus, take whatever action presents itself, and be persistent (some things take time).

I would do away with questions like "What's wrong with me?" or "Why can't I find someone to love me?" and so on. Your mind will find an answer to any question you give it, including these disempowering questions.

Learn to say "How can I...?" when you don't know what to do, instead of "I can't," and (if you are persistent in asking) you will receive the answer, every time. Learn to be conscious in what you focus on and your whole life will change.

This all may seem very utopian to you, or overly simplistic, or like a lot of work. I assure you it is not utopian (it's the way all successful people think), it IS simple, but not simplistic, and yes, it is work, at first. The great Napoleon Hill, who spent over 60 years studying the most effective and most successful people of the 20th century, concluded that -- without exception -- "whatever the mind can conceive and believe, it can achieve." He at first suspected there had to be exceptions, but toward the end of his life he said he had to admit he had not found ANY.

Let's go over that again: "Whatever the mind can conceive and believe it can achieve."

It will take some time to learn how to consciously focus your mind. It will require some effort. You will fail many times, and it will seem difficult. But at a certain point you will "get it" and at that point it will become as automatic as the unconscious focusing you have been doing. When that happens, a whole new universe of power will open to you.

More on Focusing

"And be not conformed to this age, but be transformed by the renewing of your mind, in order to prove by you what is the good and pleasing and perfect will of God."

The one thing in your life you can command is your own mind. Whatever negative people and situations you face, you can always choose a positive attitude. But doing so requires a firm, strong commitment.

Helpful: Begin by writing a self-convincing creed – I believe I can direct and control my emotions, intellect and habits with the intention of developing a positive mental attitude. Post it where you'll see it when you get up in the morning. Read it during the day, and say it aloud. Speaking an intention reinforces it. Choose a "self-motivator" – a meaningful phrase tailored to help you reach your positive thinking goals. Examples:

- Counter discouragement with the phrase "Every problem contains the seed of its own solution."

- Fight procrastination with "Do it now."

Keep your self-motivators nearby – in your pocket or on your desk – and repeat them throughout the day to instill these important new values.

Develop A Life Plan. Setting short and long-term goals each day creates a road map for your life. But only set GOOD goals!!! What is a good goal? One where you are 100% in control and one that is founded in love! A goal of raising good, healthy and prosperous children is a bad goal because you are not in control of what your kids choose. See the important difference? The goal is noble but it is not a good goal.

You identify where you're going, focus your mind on getting there and avoid many wrong turns.

Helpful: Use the D-E-S-I-R-E formula as a goal-setting guideline…

- **D**etermine what you want. Be exact, and express the goal positively. Say what you want to be or do rather than what you don't want.

- **E**valuate what you'll give in return. How much work will you do to turn your plan into action?

- **S**et a date for your goal. Be realistic, allowing enough time without postponing it too long.

- **I**dentify a step by step plan. Devise immediate, small steps to get started.

- **R**epeat your plan in writing.

- **E**ach and every day, morning and evening, read your plan aloud as you picture yourself already having achieved your goals.

Writing out your daily goals helps maintain your motivation. Keep them in your pocket or purse to read frequently throughout the day.

The Power of Visualization
Because visual images reach into our deepest mental levels, I have found pictures to be profound motivational tools. Why? Remember the mind holds everything as pictures!

Helpful: Make a list of personal qualities you want to develop…write down the names of people with whom you would like to have better relationships. Now clip pictures from magazines and newspapers that symbolize your goals.

Example: If generosity is your chosen quality, you could use a photo of someone with an outstretched hand.

Put the pictures where you'll see them everyday...and believe that you will get what you have visualized. You may also create your own "mental pictures" to defeat negative thoughts, such as dwelling on past reversals. Maintain A Positive Focus. Giving yourself positive experiences actually reinforces your positive attitude. Examples...

- Treat your five senses every day. Listen to your favorite music, taste a food you love, enjoy a beautiful view, etc.

- Cultivate a sense of humor. Laughter relaxes tension, and seeing the funny side of things helps you take yourself less seriously.

- Smile when you feel like frowning. Smile at yourself in the mirror. If this makes you laugh at yourself, the smile will be that much more real.

Now realize the optimistic face you show the world creates positive thoughts about you in everyone you meet.

How to Train Your Subconscious Mind
Did you know that often the difference between success and failure is the ability to train your mind to focus on achieving your goals and not focus on problems? It's been proven by researchers and by some of the most successful people in the world.

Getting your mind to focus and concentrate on success - so that it finds solutions instead of focusing on the problems is usually the difference between success and failure. But how do you do this?

I'm about to show you how. I'll outline the importance of training your mind, how to start directing your subconscious mind, and how to keep your mind focused so that you constantly achieve your goals and live the life you want. Disciplining your mind so that it is focused on your goals is crucial to your success. If your mind is not trained to focus on and achieve your goals then you really have little chance of success. Your conscious mind is a direct link to your subconscious mind.

So if your mind is focused on your goals and is trained to achieve those goals then your subconscious mind will also be focused on those goals and will attract the situations and opportunities for you to achieve the success you want. It's really that simple.

The minute you get distracted for a prolonged period - you lose sight of your objective and fail to accomplish those goals. In order for to enjoy success - the mind has to be regularly focused on your goals - you can't stay focused for short bursts and expect to get results.

Think of it this way, your riding in a car driven by your personal driver and every time your driver asks you where you want to go you simply say: "I don't know. Wherever you want to go is fine with me." Then when your driver takes you to the place of his choice you complain and say: "I don't want to be here, take me somewhere else." And again you say you don't know where you want to go.

Can you see the confusion you would create? Can you see how you would never get to where you want to go because you haven't trained your driver to automatically take you where you want to go? You haven't given him the proper instructions.

Your mind and subconscious mind work the same way. If you don't train your mind to focus on your goals then your subconscious mind cannot create the situations that will help you achieve those goals. When you keep changing your mind, when you are not clear on what you want - your subconscious gets confused - and you end up exactly where you don't want to be.

Let's go back to the example of your personal driver. Wouldn't it be a lot easier and more comfortable if you told your driver where you wanted to go - or even better - your driver knew where you wanted to go ahead of time? But that will only happen when you train your driver by repeatedly telling him where you want to go on a regular basis.

Your subconscious mind is your driver. Your subconscious gets its instructions from your thoughts and beliefs. Give your subconscious the right instructions and it will take you where ever you want to go in life. When your mind is focused on your goals you direct your subconscious to create opportunities for you to achieve your goals. Your responsibility is to follow up on these opportunities.

How You Can Train Your Mind
Believe it or not I get a lot of calls and emails everyday from people who want to achieve their goals but simply can't get their mind to focus on the tasks that need to be done to have the success that they want. This happens

because the mind is simply not used to focusing on your goals and following up with completing those tasks. So how do you get your mind to change? How do you train your mind?

The first step is to get the mind to stop doing what it is used to doing - or break the pattern that you've been following for so long. This will require some effort - but the reward will allow you to live the life you want and enjoy the level of success that you want.

To re-train your mind and direct your subconscious mind you start by paying more attention - so that when you see yourself getting distracted and not following up on things that you wanted to do - you take a step to break the pattern. You can break the pattern by doing something else. For example: you can start following up on what you had planned to do, you can create a list and follow up with it regularly to see if you are on track.

One thing that always works is to think about your goals every morning. As you're in bed, think about your goals and think about what you can do to achieve them during the day. If you find that you constantly say: "I don't know what do to do to achieve my goals." Then you're not looking for answers in the right place.

Take a look at what other people have done to achieve similar goals and see if you can follow the same process. For example: If you want to make more money take a look at someone else who has made a lot of money and see what they've done. Can you follow their process? Maybe you can even talk to them about the process? If you want to meet someone and be in a healthy relationship, talk to a friend who is in a successful relationship and find out what they did. By doing the above exercises you train your mind to focus on finding solutions while at the same time you direct your subconscious mind to create the opportunities for you to succeed. And - you begin to create a new pattern of thinking and you start to train the mind to work differently. You're now telling your driver where you want to go. This eliminates the confusion and allows you to achieve your goals.

You're not going to magically get your mind to focus or concentrate without you taking some form of action. When you finally do take some action your mind will still resist - but as you continue taking action the resistance will subside - REPITITION. So what action can you take? First start with the exercise I just outlined above. Next - meditate. Meditation is one of the best ways to relax and calm your mind while training it to focus on what you want. When you meditate you actually start to clear the clutter that dominates your mind.

Make the Time
Finally it seems a lot of people have come to believe that they just don't have the time to achieve their goals. If you are one of the many who have such a belief then you've really convinced yourself that your goals are not worthy of your time; because if they were you would make the time for them. I'm not talking about spending an entire day or even a few hours. It's only a few minutes at different intervals. Why try to get everything crammed into one hour? Why not try to think about your goals at different intervals during the day? For example: you may have a few minutes while you're taking a walk - think of your achieving your goals. You could also do this while you're taking a shower, driving, walking, anytime. Here's a suggestion; the next time you are driving or taking a

41

shower, pay attention to your thoughts. Are these thoughts actually working for your or against you? Would it be better to focus on your goals or keep recycling the negative clutter or junk in your head? The choice is yours - and taking action is really about taking a small step. You don't need to spend hours meditating. Even if you simply mediated for 5 or 10 minutes a day you'd be able to increase your ability to concentrate and focus by a 100-percent within a matter of days! Do it for weeks or months and you'll have dramatic results!

How to Put Your Mind to Sleep Quickly and Rest Completely

If you often lay awake, unable to put your mind to rest while you're tossing and turning, you're going to love what you're about to read, because I'm about to share with you one of the most powerful methods for quickly shutting off your mind, and drifting off to sleep.

As you may already know, your mind must be in the Alpha brain-wave stage to fall asleep. This is the stage your mind enters you're still conscious, but your body and begin to relax. It enables your more rampant and conscious mind to turn off as you enter the realm of sleep. We all know how it feels... when you're lying awake in bed trying to fall asleep, it seems like your mind is running on hyper-speed. It's almost like you're thinking 10 times faster than when you're just normally awake and alert. In fact, if you experience this often, I can tell you for a fact that your mind IS working harder than it is when you're not trying to fall asleep, and there is a very good reason for it, here's why this happens. In my books and articles on sleep, I often teach a principle: "What you focus on expands." You see, your mind responds to

42

focus, and it goes hand in hand with the law of momentum. What is the law of momentum? Quite simply:

"Energy in motion, tends to STAY in motion"

"Energy stopped, tends to STAY stopped"

In other words, if you take action in your life, and begin to create success, you will experience more and more success every day. Success breeds success. On the other hand, if you sit your butt down on the couch to watch TV and say, "Aww, just one show, I'll only watch one show," very soon you'll be sitting there for four hours, and you'll watch five or six shows.

The law of momentum is everywhere in life, in physics, with your body, and most importantly, with your "thoughts." You see, your thinking is very predictable; it all works on the law of focus and momentum. Your mind is like a big ball of potential thinking energy, just waiting for you to give it a direction to think wildly into. It awaits and responds your every command. It's an exceptional tool except, most of us aren't very experienced at "controlling" this amazing tool. In fact, a lot people aren't even aware that they can control it! And this is where sleep problems come in.

Imagine your mind like a giant overflowing lake that's just waiting for an outlet to pour into... Slowly, when it finds an outlet, it begins with a trickle of water. That trickle turns into a stream. Then, that stream turns into a small river. Pretty soon, the small river is a giant unstoppable waterfall. Your thoughts work in the same way when you're "trying" to fall asleep.

For example, you're lying in bed, frustrated, forcing your mind to not think. "I just want to get some sleep! Stop thinking! Okay, starting now... I won't think anymore. No think... nothing. My life is nothing... If only I would finally get motivated in my job maybe I would finally create the income to start traveling instead of dealing with these problems. Problems, how can I... Ahh, I'm thinking again! Stop it!"

You get even more frustrated, and repeat the process over again in a few minutes. So how do you stop it? It's easy, you see, you can easily control your thinking, except most people aren't aware of the tools necessary! The good news is, I'm about to give you the 3-step handbook to controlling your mind. Here are the 3-universal steps that will enable you to not only stop thinking; you'll also be able to lower your brain-waves into the alpha brain-state, which will quickly let you enter sleep...

Awareness
The first step to changing anything is becoming aware that it's happening, especially if it's your mind. Pretend your mind is racing, and you finally realize that you're thinking... Most people at this stage get extremely frustrated and "try" to force the mind into submission. It doesn't work! Why? Because, what you focus on expands. The more frustrated you get, the more you're focusing on frustration, so you'll get even MORE frustration and more thinking... on and on!

So the first step is to simply become "aware" of the fact that you're thinking. Nothing more. When you notice that you're thinking, smile to yourself, and say, "I just noticed myself thinking... Interesting..." Now notice what happens inside of you when you do this... something

44

VERY profound. If "I" just noticed "myself" thinking, perhaps there are really two completely separate identities running your life? There is the "I" and there is the "self."

The "I", is the real you, the higher being, the "I" behind the mind, that runs the show, the heart, the soul, the true conscious being, the choice maker.

The "self" is the mind; if left to run the show, it will run in endless circles until the edge of insanity.

The moment you do this, the moment you become "aware" - you are no longer a slave to your mind. You have won. After you become aware... do nothing, just lay there for 3 seconds and notice how it feels to be present in who you really are, not the mind, but you, the "I" - there is a great feeling of peace behind that presence in the "I." Why? Because when you are aware like this, you're aware of the power of your choice making. You now have the power of choice.

Relaxed Focus
"What you focus on expands." Now that you have become aware of your thinking, all you have to do is "direct" your mind into a place that will bring you into a deep, deep place of relaxation. Think about it, if before your mind will relentlessly race into any direction you give it; why not pick a direction that will give you peace and restful sleep?

But, most people don't know what that direction really is. It's really easy. If you focus on anything your body does or feels subconsciously, you will begin to become more and more realized. For example your breathing, the feeling of the pillow on your head, the sounds of nature outside (unless you live in the city), the warmth of your body. These are all things that happen, yet your conscious mind doesn't think about them.

As you know, "What you focus on expands"... So what would happen if you focused on something that is happening in your "subconscious"? That's right, your conscious thinking would diminish, and your subconscious mind would begin to take over the entire process of you falling asleep! It really is that simple, and it works every-time.

The easiest one is your breathing. And I promise you if you just try this tonight, you will be shocked when you wake up in the morning: "Wow! It worked!"

Repetition
As I said, the easiest one to focus on is your breathing. In the beginning, you'll find this easier said than done. Let me walk you through it.

- Begin by taking your focus onto your breathing. Take a deep breath in. Hold it for a short while, and slowly exhale...

- Count "1"

- Breathe in again... hold it shortly, exhale slowly, and count...

- "2"

Why count? Because I guarantee you, in the very beginning, you may find it challenging to hold your focus. In fact, you'll be surprised as you may not even make it to "5" the first time. This is because your conscious ever-thinking mind will butt in and interrupt. You may randomly go off into a barrage of thoughts again. If this happens, and it very well may, what do you do?

Simply become aware, and begin focusing on your breathing again. Guess what happens? As you become aware, 2 or 3 times... your mind will give up. I guarantee you, beyond the shadow of a doubt, when you get to "10" or "15" breaths you will feel a wave of relaxation in your body. This is the silent "click" as your mind shifts from the high frequency Beta brain-waves into Alpha brain-waves. Your subconscious mind will do the rest!

The following exercise will teach you how to see and recognize things that are unworthy of attention, but still recognize that they are there. In other words, attention will be paid to it and then discarded. A filter makes you totally oblivious (no attention given to it at all) that the stimuli are there and if asked to describe the situation, the filter will cause you to omit it.

Chapter 2 – Why the Unbalanced Do What They Do

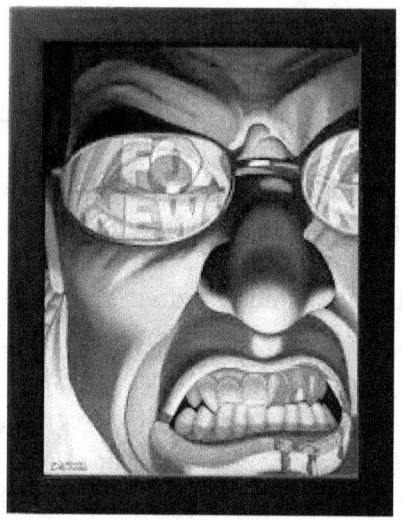

In Chapter 1, I offered a brief lesson in behavioral science. I will be relying on this information to explain why the unbalanced do what they do.

It all begins with fantasy! As a person embraces a fantasy life and chooses to live within their chosen fantasy, this fantasy life takes over as the person spirals down into the pit of depravity.

Reality has no meaning anymore; in a fantasy life the unbalanced are perfect and everything they think and do is perfect and justified.

Not all people that live within their fantasies are unbalanced or commit crimes. Many are harmless and pathetic. But the ones that have a criminal bent or radicalized nature are the ones that are most dangerous.

The unbalanced have no emotions or empathy for their fellow man. This was demonstrated by the NY Times article cited in the Introduction of this book. In the Muslim world, Islamic fanatics blow up more Muslims than non-Muslims and they simply don't care. The only meaning in an unbalanced person's life is their subjective ideology or radicalized nature and they use this as an excuse to justify their actions.

The unbalanced see themselves as different; as a person that is taking a stance. They see themselves as being smarter, more informed and more willing to right the wrongs of the world that have been committed by a plethora of evil organizations from government to religious affiliations.

The unbalanced always have an ideology that they use as an excuse to justify their actions but in reality, they will do and say anything that allows them to carry out their evil intent.

In my best-selling book, "Fantasy is Easy, Everything is Perfect," http://www.amazon.com/dp/B00BFF81CS, I delve deeply into the mind of the unbalanced person's fantasy life...

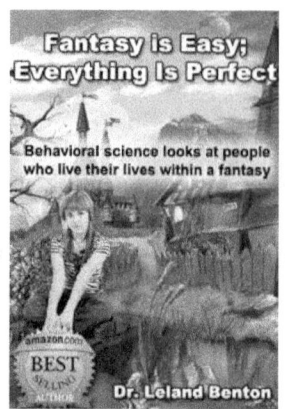

Causes of Manifested Behavior in the Unbalanced

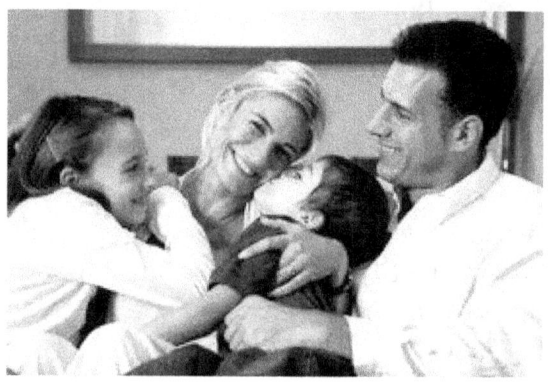

It is easy to blame mental disease for a plethora of manifested behaviors and in many cases this would be true but not always. It makes a good defense in court but many cases claiming mental incompetence are being shot down by psychologists as being shams. Many of the unbalanced are fantastic actors and will say or do anything to convince you that their cause is justified.

I want to now examine other causes of manifested behavior stemming from living a life within a fantasy.

I made a list and I will expand on this list as we go along...

- **Childhood Causes** – these are causes that develop within the course of a person's upbringing. It takes into account many of the factors listed below including childhood trauma, maturity, and environment. How we are raised, where we are raised and what type of an environment we are raised in all play a factor in a person's eventual adult existence.

- **Childhood Trauma** – a good many children suffer from many types of childhood traumas including physical and verbal abuse, molestation, bullying, disease, and more. These traumas can manifest themselves immediately or later on in adult life.

- **Child Rearing** – the way we are raised bears a good deal on how and what we become in our adult lives. Economic conditions have forced both parents into the workplace and children are left to themselves or day care facilities. The home environment contributes heavily to the problem especially if parents often fight because of finances, poor marital relations or whatever causes a tenuous home environment.

- **Maturity** – this is probably one of the most contributing factors to embracing a fantasy life since a person's maturity level bears a direct influence on how a person handles all situations in life. Remember, it is easy to be drawn into a fantasy life because everything in a fantasy life is perfect and free.

- **Mimicking Behavior Patterns** - A child that grows up in a home of violence tends to be violent. Parents that smoke and drink tend to raise children that exhibit the same behavior. Children will observe and mimic all types of behavior that they see their parents do as well as other adults and children. If left unchecked, these behavioral patterns can become set for life.

- **Environment** – the environment in which we are raised and live is the second most important factor contributing to the withdrawal into a fantasy life. It is easy to retreat into a world that the person deems as perfect. We tend to dream of the perfect but live in the flawed!! If we cannot change our physical environment then we can withdraw into a world that is far more satisfying than the one we actually live in.

- **Self-Entertainment** – this is a contributing factor that cannot be dismissed since I see it occurring almost daily. In the past, we called it daydreaming and it was deemed seemingly innocuous. Today, we now know that this trait is practiced by individuals far more often than first believed. It has become the scourge of the workplace as individuals withdraw into their own worlds leaving workloads untouched. Young people complain that the opposite gender only wants entertainment and fun with no commitment. Many complain that the opposite gender is in a world unto themselves and in many cases this is true.

- **Pathological Liars** – this is not a matter of low self-esteem; in fact it usually is a case of too much self-esteem. And more and more cases are being recorded where the individual lies but is not considered a pathological liar. Everybody lies; this is a given, but the reasons behind the lie determine the extent of which a person will go to keep his fantasy life going. In this case, the fantasy life is most important. Let me give you an example: I am going to tell you a lie right now. Ready? I am the King of France! Now you know this is a lie; France no longer has a monarchy. And I know that you know I am lying but I don't care because I am not in your world of reality; I am in my fantasy world and in my world I rule as king.

*****

It is important to note that not all fantasy is bad but to an unbalanced mind that has a propensity to embrace fantasy, it is devastating. So now let's talk about this propensity for just a moment.

It can be argued that certain individuals are born with criminal or unbalance minds. In an article I wrote years ago for a national magazine, my premise was that there are children born that are just plain evil. How can a couple have two children conceived from the same gene pool with one being good and the other being evil? I took a good deal of flack from other social scientist but not one ever disproved (falsified in science) any of my points of contention.

My Applied Mind Sciences lab, where we conduct numerous experiments on the human mind has been studying this premise for years. Our goal is to identify the area of the brain that causes criminal and unbalanced behavior.

But the fact that we as yet have not been able to identify it doesn't mean it doesn't exist. No one can deny that some people are born just plain evil and live a life filled with contention and grief.

No one can deny that these people are a drain on society and nothing society does alleviates the problem. These individuals are beyond counseling and are bent on scamming the system.

Many have no criminal intentions or are minor criminals in their actions but they share the same common trait of apathy and fantasy life where everyone else is wrong and they are right.

Chapter 3 - Are Psychological Issues a Valid Excuse for the Unbalanced?

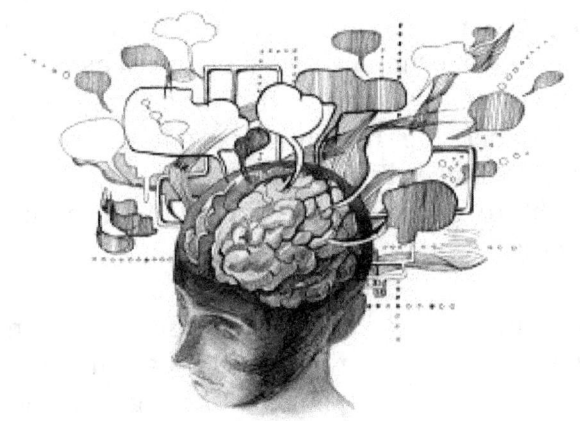

This is what I would call the "million dollar question" and it is being asked in a wide variety of circles.

On one hand you have the human rights people that claim that even the unbalanced have rights under American law.

On the other side of the equation, you have advocates that want to limit their rights to a point of actually violating American law in the interests of society at large.

The issue is a tangled mess so let's examine this for a moment.

I can easily see and I am sure you can too the validity of both sides of the argument.

America is a great country because we are a country that operates under a constitution and system of laws that govern American society. To toy or play with this system of government and laws can easily be taken advantage of by officials with hidden agendas. This has also become readily apparent on the evening news and hence; human rights advocates are highly reluctant to allow the system to be altered in any manner.

On the other hand, the government has in place special provisions for certain situations that grant executive powers that allow government to circumvent American law. For example: During World War 2, President Roosevelt actually did away with "habeas corpus" and allowed Japanese-Americans to be interned in camps with a loss of all property, etc.

It is still being argued today how government took advantage of Japanese-American citizens and abused its power. Closer to home, the debate rages on to close the prison at Guantanamo Bay, Cuba as it violates human rights.

In response, the US government has designated the prisoners at Guantanamo Bay, Cuba as war combatants and hence, they fall under military law and not US federal law.

I agree that there exists extenuating circumstances where government should be allowed special powers but there is definitely a need for close scrutiny and oversight by Congress, the Supreme Court, and with outside, independent auditors and administrators.

Furthermore, the debates still rages over the heavy handed tactics law enforcement used to hunt down the two brothers of the Boston Marathon bombings and both sides of the debate are highly committed to their beliefs.

Another raging debate is the use of public cameras that are now seemingly all over the place but were responsible for identifying the two brothers in the Boston Marathon bombing. Civil and human rights advocate argue that these cameras are totally out of control and violate American privacy rights.

One fact is certain; the various debates that range on will never go away. They will continue on all levels as well as new as the issues become known.

The question at hand, "Are Psychological Issues a Valid Excuse for the Unbalanced?" must incorporate the debates described above and I am of the knowledge and belief that each case must be taken on an individual basis since there is no way to label them all under one grouping and allow a blanket cure-all format.

"Are Psychological Issues a Valid Excuse for the Unbalanced?" is a question I want to address now.

It is my opinion that this defense has been highly abused by defense attorneys in an effort to get their clients either acquitted or a lower sentence. It has definitely been used by defense attorneys to get their clients relieved of facing the death penalty and/or capital punishment.

Here is an article that strikes very close to home on the issue being discussed....

Who Is Too Unbalanced to Be Armed?
The danger of treating gun violence as a mental health problem

Jacob Sullum | December 26, 2012

The day of Adam Lanza's murderous assault on Sandy Hook Elementary School, Mike Rogers said stricter gun control would not be an appropriate response. "The more realistic discussion," said the Republican congressman from Michigan, "is how do we target people with mental illness who use firearms?"

Last week another Republican congressman, Howard Coble of North Carolina, agreed that "it's more of a mental health problem than a gun problem right now." And last Friday, when the National Rifle Association broke its silence on the Sandy Hook massacre, the group's executive vice president, Wayne LaPierre, called for "an active national database of the mentally ill."

Psychiatrically informed policies aimed at controlling people rather than weapons are popular in the wake of mass shootings, especially among those who rightly worry that gun restrictions will unfairly burden law-abiding Americans while failing to prevent future attacks. Yet treating gun violence as "a mental health problem" presents similar dangers.

An "active national database of the mentally ill" clearly would not have stopped Lanza, who used guns legally purchased by his mother. Even if he had bought the guns himself, it appears he would have passed a background check because he did not meet the criteria for rejection.

Federal law prohibits gun ownership by anyone who "has been adjudicated as a mental defective or has been committed to any mental institution." Neither seems to have been the case with Lanza.

Acquaintances reported that Lanza might have had Asperger syndrome. That label, which soon won't even count as a mental disorder anymore, is not much more informative than saying he was a shy, socially inept loner (which people who knew him also said).

It seems safe to assume that someone who murders randomly selected first-graders is psychologically abnormal, but that is not the same as saying that a specific "mental illness" explains his behavior. Given the subjective, amorphous nature of psychiatric diagnoses, we might as well say the devil made him do it.

In any event, mental health professionals are notoriously bad at predicting which of the world's many misfits, cranks, and oddballs will become violent. "Over thirty years of commentary, judicial opinion, and scientific review argue that predictions of danger lack scientific rigor," notes University of Georgia law professor Alexander Scherr in a 2003 Hastings Law Journal article. "The sharpest critique finds that mental health professionals perform no better than chance at predicting violence, and perhaps perform even worse."

So even if the mental-health criteria for rejecting gun buyers (or for commitment) were expanded, there is little reason to think they could distinguish between future Lanzas and people who pose no threat. Survey data from the National Institute of Mental Health indicate that nearly half of all Americans qualify for a psychiatric diagnosis at some point in their lives. That's a pretty wide dragnet.

Should half of us lose our Second Amendment rights, at least for the duration of whatever mental disorder (depression, anxiety, addiction, inattentiveness, etc.) afflicts us? Assuming a prescription for Prozac, Xanax, or Adderall is not enough to disqualify someone from owning a gun, what should the standard be?

Even under current law, mental illness can become a label for unconventional political beliefs. Remember Brandon Raub, the Marine Corps veteran who was forced to undergo a psychiatric evaluation in Virginia last summer based on his conspiracy-minded, anti-government Facebook posts?

The malleability of mental illness was also apparent at a 2007 debate among the candidates for the Democratic presidential nomination. After seeing a YouTube video in which Jered Townsend of Clio, Michigan, asked about gun control and referred to his rifle as "my baby," Joseph Biden said: "If that's his baby, he needs help....I don't know that he is mentally qualified to own that gun. I'm being serious."

So perhaps excessive attachment to your guns should be grounds for taking them away. Biden, by the way, is in charge of formulating the policies the Obama administration will pursue in response to Lanza's horrifying crimes.

*****

Again, it is easy to agree with many points of the article while at the same time seeing validity in the opposing side's beliefs.

There is no easy answer here but one thing is certain; defense attorneys have abused the use of insanity or psychological issues as a defense and the psychologist community cannot agree on anything as it relates to manifested criminal behavior being a result of concise psychological issues.

Time and time again, both prosecutor and defense attorneys can easily produce psychologists that agree with their presentation of facts. They actually contradict each other.

So the debates rage on...

Chapter 4 – How to Spot an Unbalanced Person

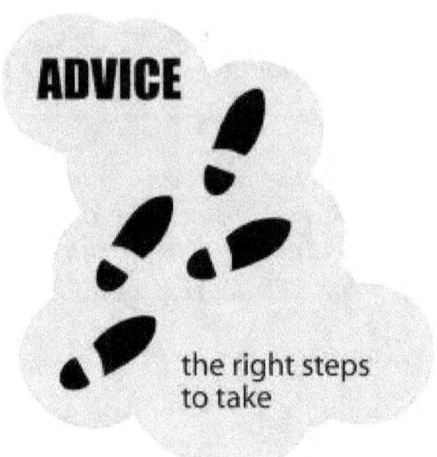

Learning to spot an unbalanced person is not as easily as it may appear. It is not a matter of spotting someone foaming at the mouth and making violent gestures and/or threats.

In fact, I can guarantee that within your own community and neighborhood there exists "ticking time bombs" of individuals waiting to explode.

Secrets, lies and tricks are tactics many the unbalanced use to manipulate people to get what they want, oftentimes destroying their victim's lives forever. The unbalanced gain a person's confidence so they can have easy access to the victim's money, trust and friendship. To avoid being fooled by an unbalanced person, look out for the following warning signs:

Blending In

Effective unbalanced people must disguise their true motives. They try hard to look and talk like others in the community and quickly limit their contact with people within their community.

Talking the Talk
The unbalanced learn vocabulary so they sound knowledgeable in the subject they are talking about.

Dressing for Success
The unbalanced want others to believe that they are regular folks, but they work hard to come across as smooth, professional and successful.

Bringing out the Worst in You
The unbalanced often expose your negative traits such as greed, fear and insecurity. They also try and make you feel inadequate if you don't believe what they are telling you, or are asking too many questions.

Fair-Weather Friends
At the beginning, the unbalanced are very friendly and take a personal interest in you. After that, the unbalanced minimize their contact with you.

Moving Frequently
Even the best the unbalanced can only play the part for so long before people become suspicious of their behaviors and motives so the unbalanced move around a lot.

Red Flags

Keep an eye out for the following warning signs:

- Secrecy – the unbalance are highly secretive.
- The unbalance always want to be 'one of the boys' and appear normal.
- They almost NEVER talk about their ideological beliefs in public and if they do it is not because they trust you but it is a matter of ego.

Know Your Own Weaknesses

These are the characteristics and situations that the unbalanced most often exploit:

- Loneliness
- Sense of charity
- Desperation regarding money (e.g. heavily indebted, business financial problems)
- Being unhappy with your life, and a tendency to look for a "quick fix"
- Falling in love (If a new romantic interest wants you to throw in your lot with theirs.
-
-

Sociopaths use flattery and inflated credentials. They talk fast, pushing you for fast decisions.

Sooner or later, you will have a run-in with a sociopath. There are just too many of them—possibly between 3 million and 12 million sociopaths in America. And they aren't necessarily locked up in jail. Sociopaths roam through all parts of society, all areas of the country, all walks of life.

There is only one way to protect yourself from sociopaths: You must know what they are, and put your guard up when you start seeing the symptoms.

*****

My goal was to give you salient information to consider that will prevent you from being the victim of any unbalanced people.

I sincerely hope my words hold value and worth to you. If you have any questions please write to me at mailto:lee.benton@epubwealh.com

I answer all of my emails and actually quite enjoy engaging my readers.

Chapter 5 – How to Protect Yourself in Today's World

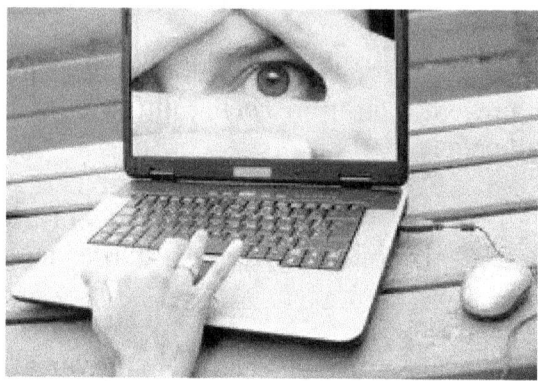

I consider this chapter to be very important but difficult since the unbalance commit a plethora of crimes.

I have included three articles below to demonstrate that protecting yourself is a varied and multi-tasking chore. Afterwards I will discuss the issues further...

How to Protect Your Health Against Toxic Behavior
http://drbenkim.com/toxic-people-behavior.html

Several years ago, I was fortunate to meet a lady named Deborah at a fasting clinic in northern California. I had several conversations with Deborah over the course of a year, and what I remember most is that her kindness was amazingly genuine - the feeling for me was that she had done a lot of inner work to identify the life principles that she strove to live by.

One day, I asked Deborah why she chose to eat her meals alone rather than with other fasting guests. After a beat of silence, she told me that she was getting some negative vibes from another guest, and that she felt that it was best for her resting experience to stay away from that energy. I remember her using the word "toxic" to describe the other guest's energy - not in a malicious way, but with a thoughtful and observational tone.

Deborah's thoughts on avoiding unnecessary toxic energy have stayed with me over the years. I feel that this facet of living is a vastly underrated determinant of health and overall quality of life. We know that our emotional health status has constant influence over the health of every organ system in our bodies, particularly our nervous and endocrine systems. And clearly, our emotional health is largely affected by our daily interactions with others. So it stands to reason that learning how to identify and effectively deal with toxic influences are important skills to develop when looking to experience optimal health.

How to Identify Human Toxicity

Generally speaking, I think it's safe to say that a person is toxic to your health if his or her behavior makes you feel bad on a regular basis. Clearly, there are exceptions to this guideline. For example, if a close friend or family member shares a concern about your behavior with a spirit of wanting to improve your relationship, you may feel bad and your sense of emotional well-being may take a temporary hit, but it doesn't make sense to label such friends or family members as being toxic.

What follows are specific patterns of behavior that I believe fall into the "toxic-to-your-health" category:

1. *Attempting to intimidate you by yelling or becoming violent in any manner (slamming a door **is** a violent act).*
2. *Consistently talking down at you, sending the message that he or she is just plain better than you.*
3. *Regularly telling you what he or she thinks is wrong with you.*
4. *Slandering others behind their backs i.e. trying to engage you in gossip that is hurtful to others.*
5. *Spending the bulk of your conversations complaining about his or her life and others.*
6. *Discouraging you from pursuing your interests and dreams.*
7. *Attempting to take advantage of your kindness and resources, and trying to make you feel guilty if you don't do what he or she wants.*

How to Deal With Toxic People and Behavior

So how do you preserve your health after you have identified a person as being toxic to your health? The answer depends on the role that the toxic person plays in your life. Although it is virtually impossible to categorize all such people into neat boxes, I tend to classify them into one of the following groups:

Group 1: H&G (Hi and Good Bye)

Examples of people who belong in this category:

Unkind customer service representatives
People who exhibit road rage
Strangers on the street

How to protect your health against such people:

1. *First, think carefully about your own behavior to see if you may have done or said something to cause the other party's behavior.*
2. *If you can identify something that you did that likely offended the other party, if possible, offer a sincere apology. If he or she accepts your apology, things work out well for both parties. If your apology is not accepted, you can at least walk away with some peace of mind, knowing that you owned up to your behavior.*
3. *If you cannot think of a single thing that you did that could have offended the other party, give him or her a silent "H&G" and walk away. Confronting the other party about unkind behavior is not likely to be fruitful. Since you don't have to co-exist on a regular basis, you can take the mindset of "fool me once, shame on you, fool me twice, shame on me." In other words, the other party's unkind behavior is on him or her; he or she will reap natural consequences in due time.*

Group 2: No real need to be close, but contact is frequent due to life circumstances

Examples of people who belong in this category:

Fellow students
Co-workers
Neighbors
Members of groups that you regularly meet with (church, book club, sports club, etc.)

How to protect your health against such people:

1. *As before, start by examining your own behavior to see if you can come up with a reasonable cause for the other party's unacceptable behavior. If you cannot come up with a reason for the other party's behavior, find someone who you can trust to be as objective and honest as possible, and explain the conflict to him or her as thoroughly and accurately as possible. Ask for honest feedback on how you might have triggered the other party's behavior.*
2. *If appropriate, apologize for your behavior. If you and your adviser have thought long and hard about the conflict and cannot identify anything that you need to apologize for, work on developing compassion for the other party.*

   Most will agree that people are not born to be mean-spirited and toxic to others. People can become mean-spirited and toxic to others for varying periods of time if they encounter enough hurt, disappointment, and/or anger in their own journeys. Maybe the other party is jealous of you and consumed by his or her own failures. Maybe

he or she is just going through a really rough time
due to a loss in the family. Maybe he or she has
never truly felt cared about by another person.
Maybe the other party has been treated so poorly
by family members that sensitivity has been
numbed and he or she has no idea that you feel
like you have been mistreated. The idea is to
generate enough compassion for the other person
to overpower or at least quell your hurt feelings.

This doesn't mean that you need to be a martyr or
a doormat and go asking for another three tight
slaps to your other cheek. Developing some
compassion for the other party's behavior is
meant to prevent said behavior from causing you
to stew and stay emotionally unbalanced for a
long time after the actual moment of conflict. And
if the other party has or develops the courage to
apologize to you, having some pre-made
compassion available in your heart improves your
chances of offering genuine forgiveness and
experiencing that much more emotional harmony.

3. *After you have worked on developing compassion*
   for the other person's circumstances, if you
   haven't received an apology, be kind, but don't
   push for a make-up session. An important part of
   experiencing emotional balance is learning to
   teach others that you expect to be treated with
   kindness and respect. To seek out a make-up
   session when you have done nothing wrong and
   the other party has not mustered up the courage

to apologize is to teach him or her that you can be walked on - not a good lesson to give.

Group 3: Ideal to be close

Examples of people who belong in this category:

Immediate family members
Relatives
Friends that you have good reason to respect

How to protect your health against such people:

1. *Go through the first two steps outlined above; try to figure out if you did something wrong, and apologize if you can think of something.*
2. *While it's important that you teach family members and close friends how you expect to be treated, in some cases, it may be necessary for you to seek out a make-up session even if the other party has not apologized for his or her behavior.*

   For example, if it was your spouse who mistreated you, and he or she has not apologized, if you know from experience that he or she is not likely to initiate a conversation that can lead to healing, and a top priority for you is to have your children grow up in a mostly peaceful and love-filled environment, it may be best for you to reach out first. By reaching out first in such a scenario, the hope is that you inspire your partner to edge closer to taking more responsibility for his or her

72

actions during the next conflict. Clearly, this proactive and almost martyr-like approach to increase understanding and intimacy is most appropriate in situations where you are deeply committed to the long term relationship at hand.

If you have any thoughts on how to effectively deal with people who may be toxic to your health, I encourage you to share them in the comments section below. Just as Deborah's behavior encouraged me several years ago, I hope that these thoughts encourage you to embrace the journey of learning how to protect yourself against toxic behavior.

I also hope that this article serves as a good reminder that we all have the capacity to engage in behavior that can be toxic to others. Staying mindful of this fact can only help to minimize the potential that we have to bring others down.

*****

How to Deal with a Mentally Ill Person: Setting Boundaries

http://angela-michelle.hubpages.com/hub/Grieving-a-Mentally-Ill-Person-the-Loss-You-Feel-When-Someone-Becomes-Ill

When someone you love becomes sick with a mental illness that refuses to get help, there are a lot of emotions that you will experience. Some of them will come right away; some of them will come slowly. One of the most surprising in severe cases is grief.

73

To someone who has not faced this, it may be hard to understand how you can grieve a living person. The terrible thing about mental illness is that the person themselves change. It's often a gradual change, from healthy to ill, but they do change. As the mental illness holds onto them, like in cases of schizophrenia, dementia, and many other mental illnesses that are gripping those we love, the person gets sicker and sicker. Unlike other illnesses, their personality changes, they may become paranoid or even volatile. One moment you are talking to the person you used to know, the next, you find them screaming at you and you don't recognize the person before you. This can happen from day to day, or even moment to moment.

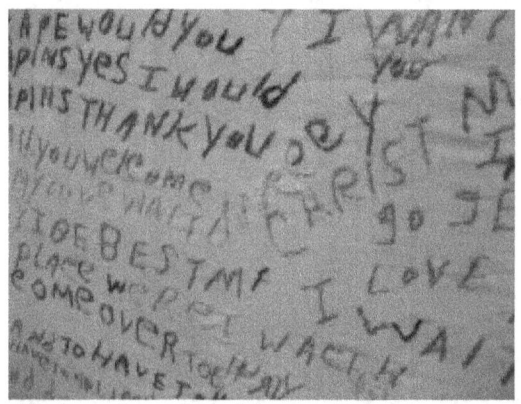

Cloth embroidered by a schizophrenia patient
Source: http://upload.wikimedia.org/

Set up Boundaries

Setting boundaries does not mean outright rejection. It means I am limiting their influence on my life. This is probably the hardest part of this kind of grief, because

74

where the boundaries should be is different for every person. The ill person may deal with certain people better than others. And different people deal with someone with mental illness more easily than others. One book I strongly recommend is called Boundaries. It teaches you that you how to set up healthy boundaries. It is not mean or heartless. It is self-preservation, love for yourself, respect for yourself. And often times it is also better and healthier for the sick person as well.

One question to ask yourself when setting up boundaries is does that person take advantage of you. If they take advantage of you, it's important for you to learn to say, "no." Until you learn to say no, they will continue to take advantage of you. You may feel you have responsibility to that person; the truth is if they are an adult, even if they are your child, you do not have a responsibility to be at their beck and call. In some cases saying, "no" is actually being more loving to that person, especially in cases of enabling.

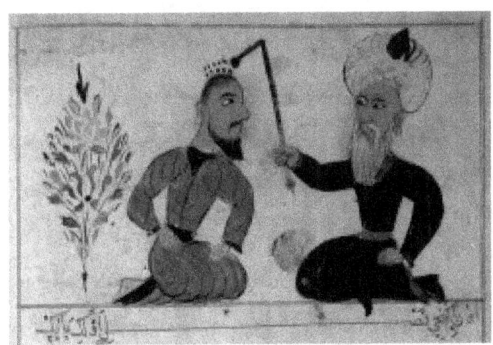

Source: http://upload.wikimedia.org/

Are You An Enabler?

That brings me to my second point are you enabling their disease? Many parents of mentally ill persons feel that they need to care for that person, even though that person is capable of caring for themselves. By setting up boundaries, you are making them take responsibility for themselves and their actions. It also teaches them to become more independent.

Another thing you need to ask yourself; is this a toxic relationship? A toxic relationship means any type of relationship where you are being abused mentally, verbally, or physically. This is the hardest kind of boundary, because for your own protection, you need to distance yourself from them. In many cases this means not allowing them in your life. Your heart will break, that's normal, but you are not only protecting yourself, but those around you. By cutting off toxic relationships it allows your other relationships to blossom.

Allow Yourself To Cry

The one thing you need to remember is you are losing someone. Maybe they are physically present in your life, but mentally the person you once loved is gone. Let yourself cry. Let yourself mourn. Remember the good times, but know that the good times you had were not with this person. It was a healthy version of this person. You can hope you will have them back, but be realistic. In most cases, unless that person seeks medical help, they will never be back. They may have moments where they are doing better than other times, but expect that things can change right back quickly.

76

Mental illness is a terrible set of diseases. There is not enough known about the human brain to cure such diseases. Although it does not take away life, it takes away quality of life. It can affect those around the ill person more drastically than any other type of illness. Be honest with yourself, be realistic, set up boundaries, and let yourself grieve.

*****

Letter Re: Dealing With Mentally Unbalanced Trespassers

http://www.survivalblog.com/2013/03/letter-re-dealing-with-mentally-unbalanced-trespassers.html

In Hearthkeeper's account of the man arrested for trespassing while attacking a chicken run, she mentions that they had decided to "press charges" as it seemed the cops were aware of the guy, but nobody else had wanted to press charges. Her rationale was that now he would get some kind of evaluation in jail.

Well, he probably won't.

I don't work in a jail environment anymore, but when I did it wasn't that long ago. What they did was well-intentioned and the right thing to do, but let's point something out...

Under every state law I've ever seen, a person who appears to be unable to care for themselves can be taken into custody for their own safety if the arresting officer witnesses the person acting in a manner that would lead the officer to believe so.

Let's examine the facts as we know them.

1. The man acted out in front of the cops

2. The homeowner wanted charges pressed

3. The cops indicated that they had had prior contacts with the guy but nobody wanted to press charges.

*So, it begs the question, **why** didn't the cops simply use their power of detention for the man's safety? I'll tell you why. They would have gotten counseled for wasting taxpayer's money and leaving their beat unnecessarily.*

*Depending on your jurisdiction and accessibility, the average time a cop will spend just processing someone "for their own good" is from 1.5 to 3 hours. Why? Because he needs to be medically cleared first. That means the cops have to take him somewhere where a **doctor** can evaluate his medical condition, the guy might actually need intervention medically and the "crazy behavior" might not just be mental illness.*

So, I take him into custody – and then I call the jail to ask them if they have a room for the guy (since I'm arresting him for a purported mental state, he cannot (by most state law) be housed with other inmates until he's evaluated. This means solitary confinement in most cases, and it means he has to be under observation 24/7 some jails set up for this by putting the person in a cell with a big window that jailers can look through, some use video cameras – but in all cases this means special treatment and you have to call the jail to see if them have the right facility.

*Next step – you think he's whacko? Are you a doctor? You can't know, so, again – before involuntarily committing someone you have to have a doctor sign off on it, the jail nurse doesn't count. Remember your reason for arresting him was for his mental state **not** that he trespassed (nobody pressed charges, remember?) In most jurisdictions this is a policy issue not a legal one, policy is set to help deal with legal issues in a fair and proper manner.*

*Mentally ill people are **not** "prisoners" in the legal sense of the word; they will have no judicial review of their case unless they are held longer than the state mandate. Anywhere they are held, they will be held **alone** – and that's resource intensive – you will have to get permission from someone to do this. So, that's the purported reason for why a cop might not arrest someone "for their own good". The biggest reason is cost. Once you've undertaken to seek treatment for this person, guess who foots the bill? The Sheriff or city that employs you.*

So, there's the Emergency Room (ER) visit for evaluation... The bill will come to your department, since once the guy is in your custody you are responsible for any medical care he may need, your status as a peace officer makes this seem easy. Your employer, however, may not see eye to eye with you on the matter. In many cases it will be impossible for you to do what's right because you will need to watch commander's specific permission, many times you'll summon the paramedics to let them "evaluate" the guy, and they will ask the guy if he wants to be treated – if he says yes, you're off the hook – because once he's in their care your hands are clean.

While you've been doing the right thing by this crazed citizen, your entire beat has been doing without you, officers who work alongside you have been doing dangerous things alone because they have no backup, in some cases calls may not be answered because policy may dictate two officers responding (like with a domestic violence case) so it's entirely possible that some wife out there is getting whacked around for a lot longer than she should be, all because you had to do the "right thing" and tie yourself up for three hours. Let's also hope you're not pushed beyond your end of shift, because overtime isn't something your supervisors like – you might need approval for that.

But let's assume we follow this guy's course after he gets a ride to the jail.

*He gets booked, just **cursorily** medically evaluated (if he's cooperative), and since it's simple trespass (a very low quality misdemeanor) after processing he'll be given a summons and released, usually within the first eight hours. Then he's back on the street. It can be quicker if the jail staff decides he's no real danger and they're overpopulated (a constant problem) and he could get released without four hours. Now he's back on the street, and he's received no medical intervention – because he's* *no longer under your control, the jail staff now makes the decision and remember, you didn't bring him in for mental evaluation, right? They absolutely will not try to create a bigger thing out of it, they'll process the trespass and release him if no bail is called for – and even IF bail is set, it's almost always a release upon personal recognizance (so you become your own bondsman). I would estimate that there's less than a ten percent chance that the jail staff will go out of their way to find this guy treatment, commonly in a setting like a jail a mentally ill person will become quiescent and not exhibit any of the behaviors that you found crazy, they're sorta in a "happy place" and don't feel very stressed – which in many cases will just make them quiet and non-threatening.*

***How** an arrest is conducted and the reasons for it are many and complex, it all boils down to dollars and cents, you'd like to think a cop is a caretaker for your community – but he's not and there are probably policies in place to keep him/her from becoming one, because it creates liability and big medical bills for the jurisdiction in question.*

*Let's not forget that now they're witnesses/victims and they'll have to go to court to testify – unless he takes a plea bargain. But guess how many times **that** happens to someone who's mentally ill? It's actually about 50/50, compared to the 95 percent plus of normal people who just take whatever is offered in way of punishment for a minor crime like trespassing. True story. Local hotel did a local homeless shelter a favor by taking in one of their "overflow" people for a night for free. Well, the guy orders a couple hundred dollars worth of room*

81

*service, and when he leaves refuses to pay. Arrest (defrauding an innkeeper) and it's revealed he's a heavily addicted bipolar heroin addict. Hotel staff gets subpoena'd. Hotel staff shows to court. Defendant is supposed to get his meds in the morning, but since he's getting transported to court he misses his morning pill and the judge continues the case because the guy isn't in the right mental state. This happens five times over a period of three months. Each time the judge sends a note to the sheriff about getting this guy his pill before ending him to court. The reason? You must be able to understand the judicial proceedings and participate in your own defense – this is **not** a competency hearing, you have no court assigned guardian. Finally seven months later the guys gets his pill, says, "yes I understand" takes a plea deal and it's over. But in the meantime five staff from the hotel have taken six half-days off to appear in court because they are subpoena'd to do so. You should be ready for this if you're going to "press charges" it can happen. It will happen.*

But let's get another thing clear, I can't speak for other states, but here's what I'd need to arrest someone in my state. The person would have had to enter into a property without permission and then refuse to leave when asked to do so. If they jumped a six foot fence to do so, and the fence was locked, then they don't get the "leave or else" thing, they can be arrested without being given the opportunity to leave. What do I mean? I mean that the cops showed up at another place under the same conditions, they should have been able to arrest him without the other parties "pressing charges" they witnessed his uninvited presence in someone's back yard

*– they didn't **need** to – but used a convenient out to stay in service "citizen declines complaint" and they move on hoping the guy wanders into someone else's jurisdiction.*

Liability for prisoners is becoming a very big headache for most communities. Putting someone in jail and keeping them there can create liabilities that get a city sued, most cities that have jails routinely pay out a couple million a year for petty complaints for mistreatment or bad conditions as the cost of doing business, we don't hear about it because there is no access to the information within a court system, and all settlements become confidential. Sheriff's have a different problem, they're elected and responsible for their own budget, reducing costs is a big thing – and if you don't have the $5,000 per patient for a 3 day mental evaluation, you're going to put a stopper in the possibility that your deputies do this.

*There is no good way to deal with mentally ill people who become violent, in many cases they don't even know they're breaking the law – having to shoot one would be something too horrible to contemplate. My advice for anybody investigating an intruder outside of your home (but still on your property) would be to not do it alone, ever. If you do decide to do it you need to do it from a far enough distance that you can retreat behind a locked barrier – bad guys can move **fast**, for most people this should just be their doorway with the screen closed and a loud voice.*

It's not a matter of you having the right to defend yourself or your property, it's a matter of never knowing

83

*if you're willing to be killed or kill someone in an unknown situation like that described. I'm pretty certain they're glad they didn't have to hurt the guy, and that the husband didn't get hurt – I've committed so many stupid-brave acts in my lifetime I know exactly how it happens, and never judge someone for doing it – but if you can plan for it better, it's always best to never do it alone and never get within running and grabbing distance of someone like that. What the police have is civil immunity for their official acts and even if it does lose them their jobs, individual cops generally don't have to pay money for what they do – we do **not** have civil liability, any act we commit against someone **may** get us sued, because as you all know – lawyers need to eat too, and sometimes it's just not convenient to put on the roller skates and snag the bumper on a speeding ambulance.*

*****

Okay, as toy can see, the task of protecting yourself is varied and wide-ranging but one thing is certain; you must become aware of your surroundings at all times.

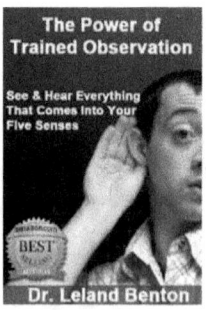

In my best-selling book that literally hit the best-seller list in less than a day, "The Power of Trained

Observation,"
http://www.amazon.com/dp/B00BSRYMGW, I offer the
following advice:

The Quiet Act of Attention

*Wendell Berry has written a poem that haunts me
frequently. As a creative writer, the act of paying
attention is both a spiritual and professional discipline.
But far too often my aspirations for paying quality
attention to everything dissolves into something more
like attention deficit disorder. As it turns out, it is quite
possible to see and not really see, to hear and not really
hear. And this is all the more ironic when my very
attempts to capture what I am seeing and hearing are
the things that prevent me from truly being present.
Berry's poem is about a man on holiday, who, trying to
seize the sights and sounds of his vacation by video
camera, manages to miss the entire thing.*

*...he stood with his camera
preserving his vacation even as he was having it
so that after he had had it he would still
have it. It would be there. With a flick
of a switch, there it would be. But he
would not be in it. He would never be in it. (1)*

*(1) Wendell Berry, "The Vacation," Selected Poems,
(Berkeley: Counterpoint, 1998), 157.*

*Just a few months ago, I went to Walgreen's for some
personal items and as I got out of my car my cell phone
rang. I answered it and was gabbing away and so before*

entering the store, I sat on the bench outside to finish my call. As I sat there a blue minivan pulled up with a woman, a man and two babies in car seats in the back. The man got out and was in the process of removing the babies from their car seats while the woman went to the back of the minivan to remove two strollers. Are you following me? A perfectly innocent family scene that should not attract any attention.

As I watched this "innocent family scene," another car pulled up with a man in it and parked alongside of the minivan. The man got out carrying a red barrel bag and saw the woman struggling with the two strollers so he went to help her. The woman thanked the man as he waved goodbye. Again, another perfectly innocent "Good Samaritan" scene but with one exception...the man had a red barrel bag when he went to help the woman but when he waved goodbye he now had a blue barrel bag. Would you have captured this observation while sitting on a bench outside of Walgreens?

I took both of their license plate numbers down and began tracking both the family and the Good Samaritan. A little over two months later I busted all three of them for heroin distribution. They never knew how we came upon them and oh, did they ask. They had the closest thing to a perfect system but it wasn't perfect enough. Trained observation always nabs the bad guys and trained observation always wins for people who use it because NOTHING gets by your five senses.

I am going to teach you trained observation and when I am finished you will be amazed at what you now see and hear that you didn't see and hear before.

In religion we have a saying, "Who is more foolish; a child afraid of the dark or a man afraid of the light?" This is an interesting statement. It goes to the heart of the matter of what do you really see, and in so doing, what do you comprehend?

What is filtered out and what is of interest to a person? What is retained and what is useful? Although the questions seem endless; the core problem is observation first and then all of the other questions fall into line.

In other words, you must first observe – see it, hear it, taste it, feel it, and smell it – before you can evaluate it with a bombardment of other questions.

This book is not about the other questions. I will leave those to the social scientists and philosophers. This book is about learning to observe with all of the five senses given to you.

It might startle you just how much information you receive daily that is filtered out completely. We will discuss filters very heavily later on in the book. It will equally startle you just how much information comes to you that is not recognized by your senses and simply "passes by". I will show you why this occurs and how to overcome the lack of observation.

Trained observation is an art form. It does not come naturally nor does it come easily. You must practice it daily until it becomes second nature and it will become second nature rather quickly if you follow my instructions. My daughters always lamented the fact that growing up with me wasn't easy because they never seemed to be able to get anything by me.

Trained observation has many attributes not only in parenting, but in business and your personal lives as well. Soon you will be able to spot the clues that will lead you to making good choices. These choices affect your quality of life so observing everything around you is most important.

C.S. Lewis once noted that if we had to choose between reading old books and new books, it should be the old books we choose. "Not because they are better," he wrote, "but because they contain precisely those truths of which our own age is neglectful."

Lewis was well aware that there were truths spoken through other worldviews that he was blinded from simply because he existed in his own.

Our worldview is no exception. Every thought and experience, every book and idea that crosses our path, has been shaped within the caldron of postmodern thought, a mindset often ruled by the eyes.

And when orientation to life is based on one's own perspective, and truth discerned by personal preference, blindness is a difficult concept to accept. But that doesn't make it less real.

Blindness is as natural to humankind as the desire to understand. We are blind to our own faults, blind to truths we don't want to hear. It is the cure to this blindness that is important.

Eugene Peterson writes, "There is widespread interest in living beyond the roles and functions handed to us by our culture. But much of it ends up as a spirituality that is shaped by terms handed out by the same culture."

What do you do to see authentically?

What do you do to protect yourself from walking blindly down paths shaped by dangerous ideas, down roads paved with misleading promises?

We shall see!

*****

My point is that the majority of readers reading this book are not situationally aware of what goes on around them and hence; they cannot protect themselves from something they cannot see or hear.

Becoming aware of everything going on around you is so vitally important in order to protect yourself from various danger situations.

I sincerely hope my words have made an impact on your lives. By learning what is contained in this book, you are better equipped to guard against the unbalanced person and his/her insidious intentions.

Now I have a special gift for you...please read on...

I Have a Special Gift for My Readers

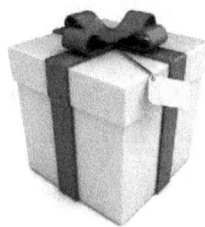

I appreciate my readers for without them I am just another author attempting to make a difference. If my book has made a favorable impression please leave me an honest review. Thank you in advance for you participation.

My readers and I have in common a passion for the written word as well as the desire to learn and grow from books.

My special offer to you is a massive ebook library that I have compiled over the years. It contains hundreds of fiction and non-fiction ebooks in Adobe Acrobat PDF format as well as the Greek classics and old literary classics too.

In fact, this library is so massive to completely download the entire library will require over 5 GBs open on your desktop.

Use the link below and scan all of the ebooks in the library. You can select the ebooks you want individually or download the entire library.

The link below does not expire after a given time period so you are free to return for more books rather than clog your desktop. And feel free to give the link to your friends who enjoy reading too.

I thank you for reading my book and hope if you are pleased that you will leave me an honest review so that I can improve my work and or write books that appeal to your interests.

Okay, here is the link…

http://tinyurl.com/special-readers-promo

PS: If you wish to reach me personally for any reason you may simply write to mailto:support@epubwealth.com.

I answer all of my emails so rest assured I will respond.

Meet the Author

Dr. Leland Benton is Director of Applied Web Info, a holding company for ePubWealth.com, a leading ePublisher company based in Utah. With over 21,000 resellers in over 22-countries, ePubWealth.com is a leader in ePublishing, book promotion, and ebook marketing.

As the creator and author of "The ePubWealth Program," Leland teaches up-and-coming authors the ins-and-outs of today's ePublishing world. He has assisted hundreds of authors make it big in the ePublishing world.

Leland also created a series of external book promotion programs and teaches authors how to promote their books using external marketing sources.

Leland is also the Managing Director of Applied Mind Sciences, the company's mind research unit and Chief Forensics Investigator for the company's ForensicsNation unit. He is active in privacy rights through the company's PrivacyNations unit and is an expert in survival planning and disaster relief through the company's SurvivalNations unit.

Leland resides in Southern Utah.

Visit some of his websites
http://appliedmindsciences.com/
http://appliedwebinfo.com/
http://BoolbuilderPLUS.com

http://embarrassingproblemsfix.com/
http://www.epubwealth.com/
http://forensicsnation.com/
http://neternatives.com/
http://privacynations.com/
http://survivalnations.com/
http://thebentonkitchen.com
http://theolegions.org

www.ingramcontent.com/pod-product-compliance
Lightning Source LLC
Chambersburg PA
CBHW070801290526
45795CB00002B/587